Flat Belly Book

Recipes Included

By Ginger Rose Gerred

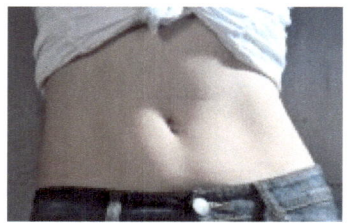

Dedicated to all those who are pursuing
health & a happier way of life

We have left room on some pages for you to make special notes.

And some images and free space in the recipe section of this book for you to keep a journal on special tips on what is most beneficial to you.

Or for you to write in your own special recipes that may not be in this book.

Chapter One
Never Say "Diet"

I have never liked the word "Diet" because my mothers friend was always on one and she was always fat. In this book I describe how I went from a unhealthy lifestyle to a healthy lifestyle while shedding almost a total of 80 pds.

The word lifestyle is a much better choice in place of Diet. Our Goal in this book is of course a "Flat Belly" and we will be targeting that from many different areas.

First we will approach this battle of the bulge through the area of health. We will come at this from an angle and goal to improve our quality of life by improving our health.

Our Goal behind the goal will always be health. That way we do not feel pressured and we can be sure that our best interest is always priority!

Make sure you check with your doctor on adding any new supplements to you lifestyle that may be mentioned in this book . Also check with your health care provider to make sure that you are able to do the physical activity described in this book. Most of them are safe and easy (for most) and physical activity will be helpful in reaching our flat belly & good health goal.

Sometimes with age our hormones can get out of balance so there will be a section of this book that will be addressing only people who have entered the mid life age bracket or pre and postmenopausal stages of their lives.

For me, that was the most difficult time of physical stress and health challenges that I faced until I corrected it using all natural supplements.

We will also be discussing the digestion process as it relates to celiac disease, vegetarians, or meat eaters and the problems that can sometimes be associated with those lifestyles.

This book will include simple steps that will become a regular part of your lifestyle and will enable you to continue to lose up to 5 pounds per month as long as you like.

Let's begin by thinking of yourself as you would think of the motor in your vehicle or the chain and mechanics (wheels, brakes, lights, air in tires, gears) on your bike which ever describes your mode of transportation.

Vehicles of all sorts must be maintained regularly or they become dysfunctional or of no use. In a car, we must change the oil every 3-4 months. They have to have tune ups and maintenance checks for the air, the water and so forth.

Our bodies also need to have our oil changed (so to speak) and we will do that by detoxifying our lifestyles. We will eliminate all white breads, white sugars, and white rice out of our food intake. And you can replace it with dark grains such as whole wheat or Udi's Bread if you have Celiac Disease.

With the exception of Xylitol which looks like, tastes like and acts like white sugar but it has Ten "10" calories per teaspoon and Zero "0" grams of fat. And is actually healthy for you and promotes clean teeth and fresh breath. While it also helps to prevent colds and flu virus'.

I substitute all sweeteners in coffee, and tea with honey, xylitol. And I substitute all food recipes with applesauce, honey or xylitol instead of white sugar. I sometimes use Xylitol or Honey in place of the applesauce when It is more suitable for a specific recipe. I found out applesauce does not work well in all baking recipes.

I Removed ALL vegetable oil out of my lifestyle and I replacing it with Safflower oil, coconut oil, olive oil, or grapeseed oil on my baked potatoes, popcorn. I did the same for all my recipes.

Refrain from purchasing any items that were produced with or by using vegetable oil. And remove them promptly out of your pantries and donate them to charity or dispose of them in the garbage disposal.

I removed all canned and bottled soda's and cola's out of my life as soon as I heard about 1 teaspoon of sugar shutting down the immune system for eight hours. I have learned how to make my own recipes for ginger ale and root beer which I will include in this book

I take all of the following supplements, vitamins, or minerals exactly as it directs on the labels of the brand that I purchase.

Cromium Picolinate taken as soon as I awaken or 30 minutes before breakfast will erases my appetite. Chromium Picolinate has also been found to combat diabetes.

Prickly Pear Cactus gives me the maximum benefits of speeding up my metabolism and also reduces my appetite.

My mother was the first person who told me about Lecithin, Kelp, B-6 & Cider Vinegar She was a smart cookie!

Recently I learned about Calcium Pyruvate. And how it attacks fat cells by breaking them down causing the fat to spit out the fat so that it will be removed out of our system.

[Borage Oil](#) also attacks fat and is so healthy for the whole body!

And for the Kicker that really tackles the fat on the belly in the form of a supplement is none other than [CLA](#) (Do Not take with Chitisan Products) CLA is derived from Safflower oil and it is my personal favorite weapon that I wage in the battle of the bulge!

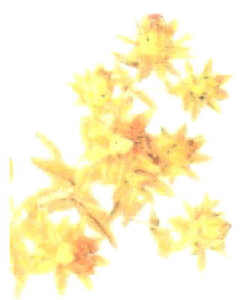

Chapter Two
Hormones & Belly Fat

For those of us who have started up the mountain our hormones may have got a little off kilter. These amino acids and supplements have helped regulate my hormones while significantly decreasing my appetite and increasing my metabolism by restoring my youthful functions naturally.

I first learned of these appetite controlling and brain healing nutrients by Dr. Eric Braverman of Path Med.

L Tyrosine

DL-Phenylalanine

L Glutamine

Pregnenolone

L-Carnosine

DMAE

DHEA

Citicoline

L-Carnitine

L-Arginine

Gaba

Lecithin

Check out Dr. Eric Braverman's free Age Print Quiz that tells your true age according to your health when you click here

Chapter 3
Celiac Disease

For those who suffer with Celiac Disease there really is no way around it other than STAY AWAY FROM "G" seriously!

But what I can tell you what I do to help heal from the damages of intestinal inflammation that it causes. I take all natural anti inflammatory supplements to help reduce the inflammation caused by Celiac Disease.

To Get rid of the inflammation:

Ginger

Turmeric

Boswellia

Willow Bark or Aspirin

Black Strap Molasses

To Aid The Digestive Process:

Licorice

Charcoal

Bromelain

Apple Pectin

Papaya Enzyme

I stopped eating all pork and most all meat in early 2001 at my doctors suggestion. But I still craved meat and I couldn't quit all together.

I will have a hamburger about three or four times a year. And I eat Chicken, turkey or fish less than twenty times a year.

After finding that I had much more serious health problems due to poor digestion after consuming meat, I began taking my food intake much more seriously.

My body has a very hard time digesting most breads, and most all meats unless I am absolutely ravished with hunger then I can digest the meat a little better. However, most breads and grains are a bird of a different color because I don't digest them too well at all.

Part of it may be Celiac Disease though I have never been tested for any food allergies. I only know I swell up like a balloon after consuming most bread types and even some grains.

My thoughts are to stay away from those dangerous type trouble foods anyway but I know how hard that is when the traditional American Diet is meat and bread.

Chapter Four
Flat Belly Lifestyle Recipes

Cola's Or Soda Pops

Ginger Ale

1 eight ounce glass of chilled soda water

1 teaspoon of ground ginger

1 teaspoon of lemon juice,

1 teaspoon of lime juice

Sweeten to your preferred taste with xylitol or honey.

Mix well and enjoy!

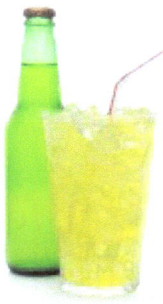

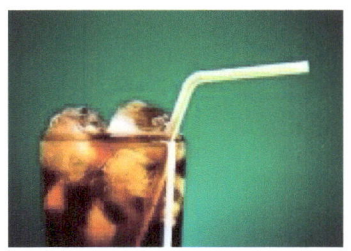

Root beer

1 eight ounce glass of chilled soda water

1 teaspoon of Sassafras

Sweeten with Xylitol or Honey

Serve over ice with a straw.

Lemon Aid

1 eight ounce glass of chilled water

The Juice of one whole lemon

Sweeten with Xylitol or Honey

Serve over Ice with a Straw

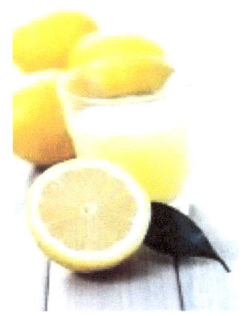

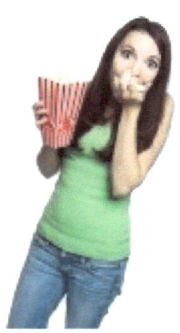

Popcorn

For healthy Popcorn that tastes better than the Movie Theater popcorn then follow this recipe:

In a medium size pan coat the bottom lightly with coconut oil. Bring it to a warm temperature. Then Coat the bottom of the pan with one layer of popcorn kernels. Place lid on it and bring it to a medium heat. Let it pop all the kernels until you hear 2-3 seconds between each pop. Remove the lid, coat cooked popcorn with ex Virgin Olive oil as generously as you like (tastes & smells like melted butter,) then lightly apply sea salt if you need to.

If you have to have a snack before bedtime Dr. Oz says that popcorn is the least fattening and most healthy snack to choose. Personally, popcorn is my favorite snack all through out the day.

Breakfast Smoothie or Meal Replacement Shake:

In a blender add 2 cups of ice

1 fresh or frozen banana

1 tablespoon of raisins,

1 tablespoon of coconut flakes

1 tablespoon of semi sweet chocolate chips

1 tablespoon of crunchy peanut butter

5 almonds

1 teaspoon of nutmeg

1 tablespoon of canned pumpkin (no sugar added)

1 store bought raw egg

1 tablespoon of milk

Mix thoroughly and serve in a glass with a straw.

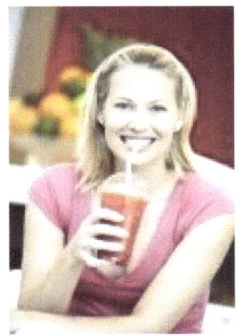

Beet Salad

3 boiled beets

1/3 cup of juice off of the boiled beets

1/3 cup of raw cabbage

3 cloves of garlic

1/3 cup of raw onion chopped finely in a food processor

3 boiled eggs finely chopped

2 avocado's chopped in bite size pieces

Keep Refrigerated until consumed

Stores for one week in the Refrigerator

 Top over romaine lettuce and Spinach salad

Top with Dried Soy or with Tofu Finely chopped

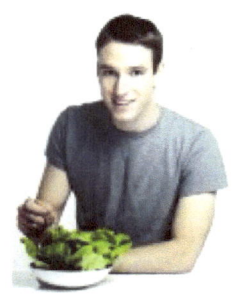

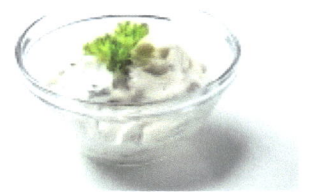

Salad Dressing:

1 cup of Plain Greek Yogurt

2 minced cloves of garlic

¼ cup of finely chopped onion

1 teaspoon of thyme

1 teaspoon of basil

1 teaspoon of parsley

1 teaspoon of lemon zest

1 teaspoon lemon juice

1 teaspoon crushed chili peppers

1 teaspoon of cayenne pepper

¼ cup of apple cider vinegar

Mix in a blender and keep refrigerated until consumed
Stores for one week.

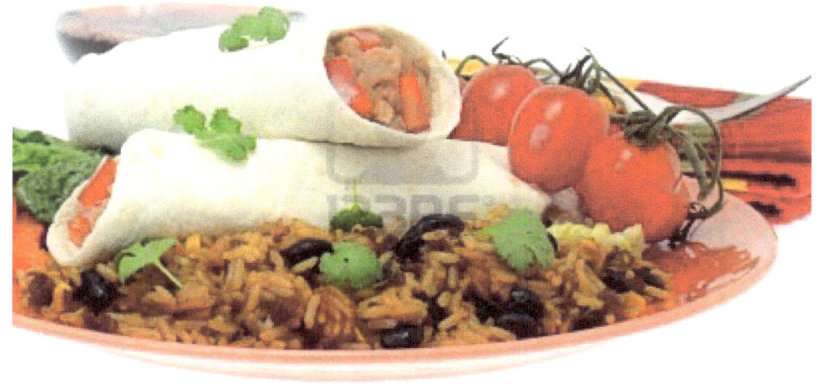

Refried Beans

2 lbs of Pinto Beans

1 onion

3 cloves of garlic

2 tablespoons of Thyme

2 tablespoons of Fennel

2 tablespoons of Fenugreek

2 tablespoons of Oregano

Cook beans till they are almost done then add the onion, the garlic and spices.

Let the beans cool, then puree them in a food processor. Serve with White Corn chips or as topping over salads or inside of a soft burrito.

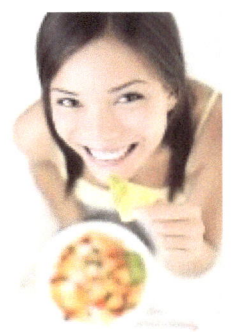

Salsa

4 cups of diced tomatoes

½ cup of minced onion

3 cloves of finely minced garlic

1 dash of cayenne pepper

1 teaspoon chili peppers

3 teaspoons of Chili Powder

1 teaspoon of chilies

1 teaspoon of lemon juice

1 tablespoon of honey or xylitol

1 can of cooked yellow corn

Serve with Chips, over Taco Salad, over burrito's or taco's

(This salsa has been medically proven to boost metabolism)

Chapter Five
Flat Belly Exercises

We are going to be working mostly on the core. However, to do it much more effective it will require some cardio vascular workouts as well.

Some of you may not be able to go jog through the park and I totally understand. And you may not even have a pool to go do laps in.

However there are YMCA's in almost every city and suburb around the nation and they will be more than happy to meet you half way In almost any given situation including financial hardships as they have programs that work with your income in most facilities.

A Stationary bike is real good for people who have knee or foot problems. The pool works even better for that. And I recommend at least 30 minutes a day of any of cardio vascular work outs which would include the following:

Again, check with your doctor before doing any of these.

Walking

Jogging

Swimming

Biking

Hiking

And to work on the core there are a few ways that we can do that. Some of them you can literally do almost anywhere you are. Others will require a flat surface to lay down on.

First of all we begin by finding your core muscles. To do so suck your belly button to the back of your spine by pulling it inward. Those are your core muscles. If you do that and keep holding in it for a count of 100 and then release it & rest for 1 min. Do that 5-10 times through out the day where ever you are sitting or standing you will begin to notice much more strength in your lower back and your posture will begin to naturally align better.

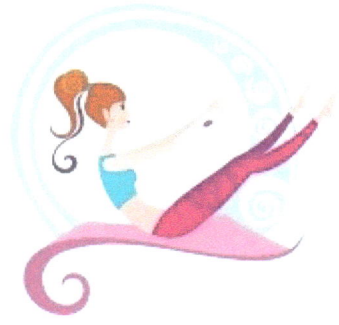

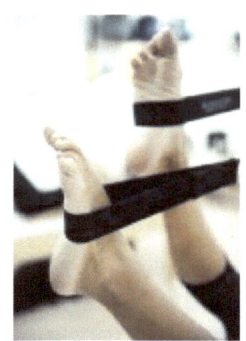

You will need a band for this exercise

Now find a place in your home where you will be comfortable and where it will be easy for you to lay on your back on a flat surface (it can be your bed as long as your bed does not swallow you when you get in it) and It must be a solid surface not a water bed.

Now reach with your hand and wrap the band around one foot. Tighten your core muscles and hold them while gently pulling your head up toward your foot. The other foot is relaxed on the bed or bent at the knee with the foot on the bed. When you have reached as far as you can go then count to 100 then slowly walk yourself back down the band to the flat position.

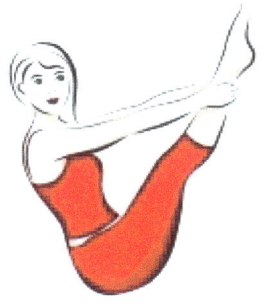